Reach Your

Weight Loss

Goals

How to lose weight and

keep it off

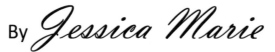

By *Jessica Marie*

Weight Loss & Fitness Coach

www.jessicamarieeenergy.com

Cover Image: RambergMediaImages

This book is a guide only and does not intend to diagnose or replace the care of your healthcare provider. Rather, it is intended to help you make informed decisions about your health in cooperation with your healthcare professional for optimal weight loss and health. You should consult your physician and get medical clearance before participating in a vigorous exercise program and/or changing your nutrition program. Specifically you should ask your physician if there are any limitations to the following: change in diet, participation in physical activity.

The author and publisher specifically disclaim all responsibility for any liability, loss, or risk, personal or otherwise, that is incurred as a consequence, directly or indirectly, of the use and application of any of the content in this book.

Table of Contents

Forward

I had struggled with my weight my whole life; even as a child I was far into the overweight category. I spent most of my life hiding and avoiding what I loved because of my weight. I always told myself I was too fat, too ugly, not good enough, too tired, or any other negative thought that you can think up, I have thought it. I did not know anything beyond these thoughts; I did not think I would ever be able to lose the weight.

I had been on diets before, and had been told to do this, or this, and not this to get me where I wanted to be. I discovered many myths and truths to some of what I had been told. I had a hard time believing in myself at this point, or even believing that I was meant to be skinny. I truly felt I was destined to be fat forever. I didn't do so well.

I embarked on one more weight loss journey. I spent the time to do my own research, break through the myths and find what truly worked for me. Through a loss of 120 pounds of fat I discovered which secrets worked best and now I'm passing on my study and research so, you too, can have success at weight loss.

Introduction

No doubt like so many others, you struggle to lose weight. Being one of the largest markets out there, there are countless weight loss products, programs and equipment to be had. How much money have you wasted on them? And what really works?

Are you frustrated and fed up with all the methods, diets and pills you have tried? Don't make your weight loss more complicated than it is, and don't be down on yourself for failing in the past. There is a way – you can lose the weight!

With our busy lives, and more and more technology being introduced all the time along with the conveniences of fast food, it sure is hard to stay active and eat a healthy, balanced diet. But if you know how to do it, it can be done, even with a busy lifestyle. Everyone is busy in their own way, so there has to be a way for everyone, right?

As you may have figured out, weight loss and staying fit are eternally linked. The less active you are, the easier it is to gain weight, especially as you grow older. But when you are active and you have a raised metabolism, you may just start losing the weight without even realizing it at first.

We are going to look at all the reasons why we gain weight, who we need to talk to when we decide we are ready to lose the weight, why keeping yourself on a schedule actually helps you to lose the weight, weight loss secrets, plus many other subjects that will help you to learn how to finally take the weight off and keep it off – once and for all!

Why We Gain Weight

We eat more calories than what our body needs in a day, so the excess gets stored as fat. Our bodies are designed in such a way, that in times when it was harder to get food, our bodies could be prepared by having stored extra calories in times of plenty in the form of fat. Now, with as easy as it is to get food, a lot of people tend to overeat, and this is a severe problem that causes many to become overweight or obese.

Genes play a factor as well by setting basic parameters on the metabolic efficiency of your body. People who are overweight many times have efficient metabolisms, meaning they need fewer calories than they are actually consuming, and they store the excess as fat. You have a greater risk of being obese if one parent is overweight and an even greater risk if both parents are overweight. However, genes only determine a tendency towards a higher or lower metabolic efficiency, not what your actual body metabolism will be.

Along with genetics, your metabolic rate depends on how active you are. It is said that every ten years past our mid-twenties we lose about 10% of our metabolic rate. This is not completely based on age; instead it has to do with how our activity levels change. The more active we are, the more muscle mass we can retain, and build, which in turn leads us to being more fit and trim because muscle tissue is metabolically active while fat is not. On the other hand, if we lead a basically sedentary life, we are much more likely to be able to gain weight and lose muscle mass.

Your eating habits make a huge difference in determining your weight. Do you favor foods high in fats and sugars? Do you eat as a family or on the go? Do you allow yourself adequate time for your meals? Are you eating the proper portion sizes?

Foods high in fats and sugars
In today's busy lifestyles, we may not realize how often we are eating these foods. If you are one who is always ordering out for work, or going out to dinner as well, this is not going to keep you healthy because you do not have the control as to what is being put in your food and it is much harder to make sure you are eating the right kinds of things and getting all of your nutrients.

Watching your intake of foods high in fats and sugars is huge. We all need nutrients, including healthy fats, to keep us balanced, but eating a lot of junk food and sugary drinks will attribute greatly to us gaining more weight. Processed foods don't generally have a lot of nutrients in them, or any at all, and they are high in salt, sugar, and unhealthy fats.

Eat your meals family style
How you serve the food can dictate how much food you eat. Do you sit down at the table and serve it the food family style where everyone can share in the meal?

Eating as a family has been proven to lower the amount of food you consume. This is a great time to come closer as a family and slow down your eating time while you are discussing the day's activities. By slowing down your eating, you allow your stomach to send the proper cues to your brain that it is full.

In reality, on a scale of 1-10 of fullness, we should feel right around an 8, when we are done eating. It takes some practice, but you can learn this trick and you will feel so much better knowing you did not stuff yourself to the maximum capacity.

Watch your portion sizes

Portion size is one of the main reasons people eat too much. Over time, larger portions of food have become the norm, especially at many restaurants. Going out to eat is fine every once in a while, but be sensible in what you are choosing, and remember you don't have to clear your plate of the large servings that you are given.

Learn portion control. This is usually a huge factor for most people, and they do not realize how much they are actually eating. Your plate needs be divided fairly evenly. This means protein, starches/carbohydrates, vegetables and fruit all equal ¼ of your plate.

Eating several small meals (5-6) throughout the day, rather than two or three big ones, will also help you eat less. During the early stages of creating a healthier eating habit this can definitely keep those hunger pains away. Another really important thing is to eat your breakfast (preferably within ½ hour to 1 hour of waking up), as this sets up your metabolism for the day. If you skip breakfast, your body will begin to store more fat because it will think you are starving.

Exercise is essential to a healthy lifestyle and to maintaining a healthy weight. When you exercise, including cardiovascular training, strength training, and flexibility training into your workouts, you gain muscle mass and raise your metabolism. You in turn, begin to weigh less, look leaner and look more toned because muscle takes up less space than fat. Strength training also helps reduce the risk of accidental injury, improves your bone density, helps with digestion and helps in lowering your blood pressure, cholesterol and triglyceride levels.

As you can see, even if your family has a history of being overweight or obese, diet and exercise are the two main factors that affect your health and weight. Regular exercise and proper nutrition is essential in reaching and maintaining a healthy weight.

Creating the Perfect Weight Loss Plan

When most people think of losing weight, they think of going on a diet. Many times, this means finding some fad diet that is probably popular at the current time, and trying to follow all of its crazy rules and recipes, like lemon juice, cayenne pepper and maple syrup. Honestly, who enjoys these things? Do you like cutting out entire food groups such as carbohydrates or drinking crazy concoctions that simply do not taste very good and do not fill you up?

It is doubtful that anyone does. Yes, there are a few diet plans out there that have some merit to them, but most do more harm to you than good or make you go crazy with hunger, causing you to fail in the end anyway. This is why it is beneficial for you to change your thinking from "I'm on a diet," to "I have a healthy diet."

Fad Diets

These diets usually consist of removing one food group entirely from your diet or drinking an unusual mixture of ingredients to get you to lose weight. Not only are these unhealthy and dangerous, they can leave you feeling hungry or drained from lack of proper nutrition. In the end, even if you do lose some weight at first, these diets usually fail because they are too restrictive and as soon as you stop them you wind up gaining all the weight back, plus some.

Eating Too Little

Dieting for some people means just eating very little. If you do not follow a proper diet plan, and think that not eating is the way to lose weight, you will quickly find out that besides being very hungry you will not feel well because you are not getting enough nutrients. You are also confusing your body's metabolism with this starving method – it might not make you lose weight much at first as your body starts to store all the fat it can when you do eat. Plus, on the serious side, if you go to this extreme long enough, you will end with an expensive hospital bill rather than a healthy you.

Dieting is a huge industry, and at times people get suckered into the latest fad diets, diet pills and supplements. You need to be careful about what products you choose, or what methods you decide to use, and avoid falling for something that can cause you more harm instead of helping you live a healthy life.

With all the information out there telling you what you should or should not do, it gets very confusing. When it comes to successful, healthy weight loss there are some things that you should avoid.

Starving Yourself

Starving yourself, fasting or going on a diet with too few calories causes major health risks. Yes, you can lose weight doing these things but you are going to lose more muscle mass instead of fat and interrupt the proper functioning of your metabolism. After you have lost the weight and go back to eating normally you will gain the weight back, plus extra.

When you interrupt the proper functioning of your metabolism, it causes a shift toward increasing your risk for diabetes, metabolic syndrome and other health risks. You actually want to raise your metabolism leading to a higher percent of fat loss. Eating actually helps your metabolism when you eat the proper amount of food with high nutritional value. It is advisable that as a woman you stay at or above 1200 calories and as a man you stay at or above 1400 calories a day. When you drop below this number your body has a hard time getting all the nutrients it needs for fueling activity and satisfying your hunger.

Supplements and OTC diet pills

Taking supplements or over-the-counter diet pills is risky since it is unclear as to what their side effects are. More often than not, these products are hyped up by a lot of empty promises that do not deliver, and they cause high health risks. Although they may not appear dangerous, they are still dangerous because they are loaded with caffeine and diuretics.

Using these cause you to become dehydrated and have imbalanced electrolyte levels. These products are also huge waste of your hard-earned money. It is safest to forgo the supplements altogether and rely on eating a healthy, balanced diet (that gives you all the nutrients and minerals you need) and exercise to lose weight.

Detox and cleansing plans
Cleansing your body to get rid of toxins is totally unnecessary. Most detox and cleansing plans include diuretics which cause weight loss due to water loss. They are very dangerous and unhealthy, as well. When using a detox you run the risk of becoming dehydrated and having electrolyte imbalance among many other health risks. (Losing large amounts of water, especially on top of fasting without medical advice is very risky.) Your body is well designed to detoxify itself; forcefully cleansing it out is unnecessary.

Instead, focus on exercise and nutrition. If you really still feel the need to cleanse, use my "Natural, Healthy Cleanse" (link provided at the end of the book) which includes eating a well-balanced diet and drinking proper amounts of water.

Purging
Purging, in any form is not safe. It includes forcing yourself to vomit and abusing laxatives. These methods are

commonly seen in colleges, but they can cause very serious health conditions and are the first step in developing eating disorders.

The acid in your stomach is very strong, as it is meant to break down the food you eat. Repeatedly forcing it through your esophagus and mouth can cause erosion of the esophagus, mouth and your tooth enamel. This increases your risk for certain cancers, tooth decay and more. You will also experience dehydration and again an imbalance of electrolytes as a result of fluid loss.

Any form of purging is extremely dangerous and risky for your health; weight loss with this form of "dieting" is not a loss of fat, your weight will come back plus some once you stop. If you have a problem with this, seek medical help immediately.

Over Exercising
Extreme exercising can put you at great risk for injury, cause severe wear and tear on your body and cause dehydration and electrolyte imbalances. In some cases, over exercising causes us to psychologically turn exercise into a form of punishment for eating.

The recommended amounts of exercise vary greatly depending on the person. Choose the amount that best fits your goals and lifestyle. Some people prefer the intense workouts while others are comfortable with 30 minutes of cardio five days a week or 20 minutes vigorous cardio 3 days a week and 8-10 strength training exercises 2 days a week. Stick with what is comfortable for you and does not leave you feeling exhausted for the next 2-3 days.

Do regular exercise for all the health benefits including relief from daily stressors. Stress causes the release of cortisol which increases appetites and stimulates fat storage.

Legal or Illegal Weight Loss Drugs

Using drugs that are not intended for weight loss is a very bad idea that can be very dangerous. The risks that go along with abusing drugs such as cocaine, speed, attention deficit disorder drugs, thyroid medicine and diabetic medications for weight loss far outweigh any health benefits that you might get from the weight loss itself.

Risks include physical and psychological addiction, social and financial problems, ruining your relationships, anxiety, very bad headaches, stroke and heart, lung or kidney problems. Using any drug for purposes other than which it is intended is highly discouraged because of the potential dangers.

If you are using a weight loss medication, prescribed by your doctor, follow all the instructions, keep in constant contact with your doctor, and watch for side effects.

Tobacco

Smoking has countless health risks to begin with, yet some people actually use it for weight loss because nicotine has been shown to be an appetite suppressant. But again, the risks from smoking far outweigh any weight loss benefits, as smoking harms almost all the organs in your body.

Plus it causes cancer, cardiovascular, respiratory and other disease and reduces the health of the smoker overall. When you do quit, weight gain is generally a very common side effect.

Losing weight is about creating a healthier lifestyle for yourself, do you really want to give yourself unnecessary health risks along the way? Be aware of your choices and choose the options that will give you the healthiest benefits along with your weight loss.

When you are ready to choose your diet or eating plan, there are certain things that you must take into consideration to make sure that you are picking one that will help you to attain the weight loss goals you have and to make sure you are staying healthy. Some diets, as we mentioned, do not contain a balance of nutrition that your body needs, and can therefore make you very ill, and won't help you to lose weight properly. By using the following guidelines you can create a diet plan that is right for you.

Define Diet

A diet is the customary amount and kind of food or drink taken by a person from day to day; more narrowly, a diet planned to meet specific requirements of the individual, including or excluding certain foods.

Realistic Expectations

You must realize that losing weight takes time, and depending on how much you have to lose will depend on how long it will take you. You do not want to take on a plan that promises you will lose a lot of weight in a short amount of time (such as 10 pounds in one week), as that is most likely going to be a very unhealthy and unsafe option for you. After the initial two or three weeks when weight gain might be up because of water loss, you should be losing around 1-2 pounds a week to maintain healthy weight loss.

The Right Nutrition

Make sure you look over any diet plans you are considering thoroughly and see what they allow or suggest for you to eat. If it has a balanced-looking diet to it with the right amounts of foods from the food groups, you are probably looking at a plan that is safe. Any of the fad diets that cut out whole food groups, or make you starve yourself or drink strange concoctions are not safe. You also want the right amount of protein, carbohydrates, fiber and make sure you are getting no more than 30 percent of your calories from fat per day.

Realistic Diet Plan for You

While you are researching different diet plans, make sure it is something that will suit you and your lifestyle. If you are a very busy person who is not home a lot, look for a plan that has convenience as well as healthy choices. If you wind up choosing a plan that you don't stick to for whatever reason, you will find yourself becoming derailed from your plan and go back to your old ways and feeling worse than when you started.

Calorie Level

Make sure that the plan you choose has you eating enough calories. You essentially want to cut out enough calories so that you can lose those 1-2 pounds a week. You have to weigh this all against you and your activity levels; how many calories you need each day will vary from person to person depending on how active you are and your starting weight. You might want to work with a trained health professional to help you decide which is best for you.

The weight loss industry is not telling you everything– nor do they want you to know. Their business is booming thanks to all the fads, gadgets and pills out there that are being purchased people wanting to lose weight.

Unfortunately the only things, in most cases, that are getting lighter are the pocketbooks. Most of the fads, gadgets and pills do not work, and only a small percentage of people purchasing these items manage to lose the weight and keep it off.

I want to let you in on these secrets.

> Diets don't work…permanently! You have heard this one before; you know it's true. There are a lot of fads out there and proposed "magic bullets." The bottom line is that you need to find the lifestyle that works best for you. It's a lifestyle change and a mindset rather than a diet. It's not something that you choose to do in the summer before bathing suit season and then stop once winter rolls around so you can become a couch potato, once again, and gain all the weight back.

Your "mindset" plays more of a role than you think when it comes to losing weight. Your success weighs heavily on your mindset...after all that is something you have control over. You do not need to give into all the ads for exercise equipment and "diet pills" that are advertised on television; if you set your mind to losing weight and loving yourself then you will.

Most weight loss product ads deceive the buyer. A majority of the weight loss products you hear about on the radio and see on infomercials only do what they claim for 1 out of every 100 people. Even so, consumers are lured into buying these products with promises like "Lose the weight and keep it off", "Eat whatever you want" and "no diet or exercise required". If it sounds too good to be true, it probably is.

Just because they say it's "scientifically proven" or "doctor-endorsed" doesn't mean it works. These claims are typical on many weight loss products, but they never tell you anything about where the studies were made or by whom, avoiding the opportunity for you to check out the validity yourself. Often these health and science professionals have a financial interest in the product.

Just because the government allows a product to be on the market does not mean it does what it claims. Plus, the product can go on the market before it is officially government approved. It may not be life threatening, but do you want a product that is going to slow your metabolism down causing you to develop other health problems?

Products toted as 'natural' or 'herbal' are not guaranteed safe. People also assume that just because a product is made of natural ingredients means it must be safe as well. But until the FDA receives evidence that a product is harmful, the companies are free to put their products on the market. Along with this, only a few 'natural' or 'herbal' vitamins and pills are FDA approved.

A product only needs to work for one person for the company to make the claim. There are plenty of products that claim to do things that they just do not, and you should steer away from products making high and lofty claims.

The lose weight fast fad diets sound great, but anything that requires sudden and radical changes to your eating pattern is very difficult to sustain over time. They will send you into a quick cycle of weight loss which is always followed by a rebound period where you gain the weight back then some once you resume your "normal" eating patterns. Plus, the next time you try to take the weight off, it makes it all that much more difficult. These diets have little to no health benefits. If any one of them worked, do you really think there would be the need for more?

There is not a quick fix or magic pill that will help you lose weight. If the product is making such claims, you can just about guarantee that they will not work. Losing weight takes work; you did not put the weight on overnight, nor can you take it off overnight.

Now that you've decided you want to lose weight, you should include some other people in your weight loss journey. These people can help you with many aspects, including choosing your diet plan, setting your goals and encouraging you along the way.

A Weight Loss Coach

Every day we make choices to do or not do many things. These choices may range from profound to trivial and each one has an effect that makes our lives more fulfilling or less fulfilling, more balanced or less balanced, that makes our process of living more effective or less effective. Weight loss coaching helps you learn how to make choices that create an effective, balanced and fulfilling life. Weight loss Coaching is a profession that is profoundly different from consulting, mentoring, advice, therapy, or counseling. The coaching process addresses specific personal weight loss, fitness and nutrition goals, projects, business successes, general conditions and transitions in the client's personal life, relationships or profession by examining what is going on right now, discovering what your obstacles or challenges might be, and choosing a course of action to make your life be what you want it to be. A weight loss coach helps you discover what your own personal "best" might be. Give this a try with a free assessment call, you will begin to see your goals become a reality.

A Fitness Trainer

A lot of people may have never learned to exercise properly. A physical trainer will make sure that you do, and will push you to attain your fitness goals, and can also help set your goals. They will oversee your exercise routine in a gym, giving you both cardio and strength based exercises to follow.

The main goal of a personal trainer is to see to it that you get fit, and educate you on how to do it properly for yourself. Each person is different in their needs, and a personal trainer can adjust your training program to fit you just right. Over the course of the weight loss process, both the physical trainer and the dietician may give you advice in changing up your diet and your workout routine as you begin to gain more muscle tone to help support your new muscles.

Friends and Family

When starting your weight loss journey, let your friends and family know what you are doing so that they can be supportive of you. It always helps to have people you know and trust and that stand by your side in any endeavor.

You can even have a friend, or your spouse, keep you accountable to keep you from sneaking any extra snacks or sweets, or to keep you on your exercise regimen. You will likely be more successful in the end if you have someone come alongside you (even over the phone if they are long distance) who will help encourage you while you are reaching your goals and to help push you when you start to struggle. Then, when you do reach your final goal (or even mini goals throughout) you can celebrate your achievements with the ones you love.

A Dietician

A dietician will have a wide range of knowledge that can help you to understand your body and to help prepare a food plan that will fit your particular needs; in most states they are required to get a medical license before they can become a dietician.

Their goal is to help you eat healthier, and in turn maintain a healthy weight. Dieticians stand apart from anyone who promotes a fad diet because they are not nutritionally sound for you. A dietician will also help you figure out how many calories you need to consume in a day and balance your intake of all the food groups that you should be eating from daily.

A Therapist
Some people know they overeat, and how unhealthy it is for them as well, yet can't seem to stop their overeating no matter how hard they try. Many of these people eat for emotional reasons; whether it is hurt, sadness, boredom, happiness, anxiety, or any other emotion they relate it to food.

This is someone who should seek the counsel of a therapist or other professional trained in this specific matter so they can get the proper support. In some severe cases, it will take checking themselves into a clinic designed for this purpose so that they can be closely monitored for specific amount of time.

It is up to you as to whom you connect with. It is my strong advice that you choose, at least, one or two of the people listed above to build a strong support system. This support system is the foundation of your weight loss success, the stronger it is, the more success you will have.

The next step in planning your weight loss goals is to set up a daily schedule. Make sure you write it down. You need to decide what time is the best for you to exercise. Find a time that is going to be uninterrupted by family, meetings, shopping, daily events; this is the time when you will best stick to your routine. Mornings, before your day gets started, provide a good opportunity. You will not have an excuse to miss your workout because nothing else will be schedule yet, plus it will give you much needed energy to get through the day.

Also schedule out your meals, including the times and food you eat each day. The best thing to do is to schedule them out for a week at a time. By planning your weekly meal schedule you will be able to create a shopping list, which in turn keeps you from being tempted to impulse buy or stray off of your diet.

The next thing to schedule is "me time" (time that you spend on yourself) each day. This is when you will reflect and focus on your goals, go through your affirmations, read a book, take a hot bath, or whatever you decide you are going to do with that time. It is a time for you to be by yourself and relax without interruption so again, you want to make sure this is at a time when you will not have excuses to miss the activity.

Why is a daily schedule important? It is how you stay focused and motivated to reach your goals. With a daily schedule there is not a question about what you need to do, you can keep yourself in check and in the end you lose more weight.

Know What You Are Doing Each Day

Having a schedule allows you to be prepared ahead of time, giving you less stress and more freedom to enjoy your day. You will be able to schedule the rest of your day, or other activities that may come up, around your workout schedule, meal schedule and your precious "me time" schedule. You won't miss that workout because you accidently scheduled something else in that time slot and you will be giving your body the proper energy it needs to make it through those other activities.

Keep Yourself in Check

Giving yourself a specific schedule to follow allows you to be more likely to stick to your goals. You have a written account of how you are being successful. Keeping a journal (in a notebook or on your smartphone) specifically for this is a great way to reflect on your goals and notice where you may need to change things up. If you do miss a scheduled workout, or have an extra snack, you can keep note of it and see how it affects your weight loss.

Lose More Weight

By keeping yourself on a schedule (and writing it down), you will tend to lose more weight. You will complete more of your workouts (or miss very, very few in the long run), eat healthier meals (when you write what you eat, you are more conscious of the choices you make) and feel more relaxed because of the time you allow yourself to unwind.

How to Maintain Your Weight Loss

Once you have reached your target weight, you will need to switch to weight maintenance mode so you do not put all that hard work to waste! Educating yourself ahead of time will help you when you are at the point where you have attained your weight loss goal. You will want to celebrate your weight loss and continue with your newfound healthy lifestyle.

During your weight loss journey you created a schedule and picked up new healthy habits. You want to continue using those new habits.

Eat All of Your Meals

Remember, if you stop eating properly scheduled meals (or skip meals all together) your body's metabolism will take this as a signal that your body is starving and will begin to store fat for reserves. Make sure you keep up with eating your meals, scheduled out as you have been. Keep in mind that if you skip a meal at one point in the day, it could mean you overeat later on when you are just so hungry.

Keep Eating a Variety of Foods

This will keep you getting all the nutrients and vitamins your body needs to function properly. It will keep you feeling healthy, energized and protect your body. Make sure you continue eating whole grains, fruits, vegetables and lean proteins.

Keep Eating Frequently

Eating five to six small meals a day as you have probably already learned to do is a good thing to continue doing, as this keeps your metabolism up, and keeps you feeling satisfied. It is important to continue this way of eating because it is easy to fall back into the trap of eating larger portion sizes again if this was a problem before. You have worked so hard to reach your weight loss goal; do you want to gain your weight back?

Keep the Junk Food to a Minimum

Now that you've developed your healthy habits, why ruin it by going back to your old ways and eating all that junk food? You have discovered plenty of delicious tastes to satisfy all your cravings with healthy foods. Keep your intake of fruits and vegetables up to several servings a day, preferably 6-8.

Keep Exercising

You have gained the knowledge of what works best for you and how it affects your body. Do you want to go back to feeling tired and unhealthy again? Remember to change up your routine. Changing up your routine is a great way to keep you from getting bored, and to keep your body guessing. At this point, you may choose to cut down your exercise time. Instead of working out for an hour a day you can try a half hour a day. As long as you are always combining your cardio and strength training, you will continue to stay fit, strong and healthy, all while protecting yourself further from illnesses coupled with your healthy diet.

Adjust Your Daily Caloric Intake

Many people wonder if they should increase their daily caloric intake right away. It is probably advisable to do so, but do so gradually. Try starting with just 250 calories more a day. After a week, weigh yourself. You'll probably still have lost some more weight. If this is the case, add another 250 calories, then weight yourself a week after that. Repeat these steps until you see that your weight has remained the same when you weigh yourself for the week. If you gained a bit, take away some calories, 100 at a time, until your weight evens out and remains the same from week to week.

Keep Drinking Water

Keep drinking at least eight glasses of water a day to keep your body working well. Water aides in digestion, increases your energy and helps rid your body of toxins naturally. Plus, you will stay hydrated and healthy.

Keep eating frequently. Eating five to six small meals a day as you have probably already learned to do is a good thing to continue doing, as this keeps your metabolism up, and keeps you feeling satisfied. It is important to continue this as well because you don't want to fall into the trap of increasing your portion sizes again if this was a problem before. You will throw yourself all the way back to square one eventually. In the very least, you will gain a bunch of the weight back you worked so hard to shed.

Everybody wants to live long and healthy lives; nobody wants to count on getting any severe diseases. As humans we are unable to control, predict or prevent every situation; however, there are ways we can help protect ourselves that can make our lives more full and healthy.

Prevention and early detection

> Most people dread going for a yearly physical, or even the dentist cleaning every six months, but having good doctors and keeping these appointments in your life will help you to stay healthy because you doctor can detect things that you can't on your own.

Know your family history

> Knowing your family history is an important thing to become informed about. If there is any history of heart disease or cancers in your family, your doctor can keep any eye out for symptoms and do regular testing.

Love the people who surround you

> Make sure you spend time with the ones who surround you daily such as your spouse, children, other family members, friends and coworkers. Enjoy

the time you spend with other people, plus maintain healthy friendships. These relationships are the foundation of your weight loss support and are needed to help you feel fulfilled in life.

Get seven to nine hours of sleep

Many of us find this task difficult. We have many excuses from having to go to work or having to take care of family to just not having any time. Life can get busy, which is all the more reason to make sure you get your sleep. Getting 7-9 hours of sleep can do many things like reducing stress, give you more time in your day and make you more capable of taking care of yourself and your family.

Find time for the things you enjoy

We all have times where we need to be doing something we really enjoy and most of these are things that we excel at. When you include things that you are good at, you boost your motivation and give yourself the want to continue on your chosen path of weight loss. It is also good to spend time doing things you enjoy, as it can be soothing and help relieve stress.

Manage your stress – don't ignore it!

Everyone has stressors of some kind, and it is important that we handle our stress so that it does not get out of hand and consume us. When you are riddled with worry and stress it can literally make you sick in many different ways. Daily exercise of just 5 minutes can help clear your head, and make sure that you are not over-filling your daily agenda.

Find balance in your life

Keep your projects at work and the ones at home at a balanced point. By letting one or the other takeover you can become unmotivated, stressed and begin to throw your weight loss efforts out the window. Find a balance so you are still able to enjoy all the other things around you like your hobbies, your friends and your family.

The benefits of staying healthy are boundless. It is more than just being happy with the way you look and can fit into that new outfit. Being healthy is about you as a whole: physically and mentally.

Your Physical Health

Keeping yourself physically healthy can help you all around. Along with helping you to better be able to take part in daily activities such as walking, moving and bending, it allows you to be physically able to take care of your loved ones who depend on you.

Make sure you are eating a healthy, well balanced diet to help you improve your physical health. Keep in mind that the foods you choose to eat can have a direct impact on your health. When eating a proper diet you are giving your body very important phytochemicals which help prevent things like heart disease, specific types of cancer, diabetes and high blood pressure. They are found in foods such as berries, spinach, olives and kale. Eat a diet of lean proteins, fruits, vegetables and whole grains to help protect your cardiovascular health.

Striving to live a healthy lifestyle will help you live a long, healthy life. Even though you do not have control over all health problems, you can take control and prevent many of them from occurring.

With the leading causes of death being chronic diseases such as diabetes, heart disease, stroke and cancer, having lifestyle choices that include controlling the foods you eat, keeping your weight at a healthy level, how much you exercise and how you deal with the stressors in your life can have a huge impact on keeping these diseases from presenting themselves.

Other benefits of a healthy lifestyle include improved digestion and a lower blood pressure. Keeping yourself healthy can also help ease or eliminate back problems and back pain plus improve your posture, enhance coordination and balance, and lower your resting heart rate.

Your Mental Health
Having poor mental health also affects your physical health. When you allow yourself to be over-stressed, or for that stress to rule your life, it can make you sick.

Stress raises your blood pressure which increases your risk of a heart attack or stroke. You need to deal with your stress in positive ways through exercise, meditation or therapy. Learn to avoid using eating, drinking or smoking as stress relievers.

Living a healthy lifestyle can also improve your mood and give you greater self-esteem and mental focus. You will be stronger, have more stamina and you will be able to get a better night's sleep.

Conclusion

Now you are ready to plan and start out on your weight loss journey. As you can see, you don't need to buy into some crazy diet, machinery or drinks. There is no quick fix as many ads would like you to believe. This is about you creating a change in your lifestyle.

The best things for you to do is take charge of your health by changing things like your diet, your activity levels and keeping your mental health in check. When you take the time to assess your current lifestyle habits, sitting down with your doctor and other professionals like a weight loss coach, nutritionist and a physical trainer, you will be able to develop a weight loss treatment that is designed especially for you.

Learning as much as you can about your body and how it operates, your family health history, and how to manage your physical and mental health will help you live a long healthy, life. With as many advantages as there are to living a healthy lifestyle, if you are determined and can keep yourself motivated and focused on your goals, you will, with the proper amount of time, reach those goals. It takes hard work and determination, but you can do it!

Extras

If you enjoyed this book and found it helpful, share with others by writing a review.

If after reading this book you want more information on weight loss coaching, visit jessicamarieenergy.com or email me at jessicamarieenergy@gmail.com.

Get more information on my "Natural, Healthy Cleanse" here: http://jessicamarieenergy.com/blog/2012/08/08/natural-healthy-cleanse

About Jessica Marie

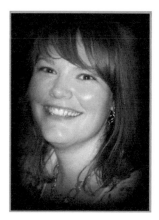

At the age of 26, after spending my entire life using the excuse "I'm big boned", I came to the horrible realization that I was 130 pounds overweight. This put me into the Extremely Obese category. I knew I had to change my habits. Through my weight loss journey of losing those 130 pounds my knowledge on how to lose weight grew and I developed a passion for helping others.

I changed my life and now I help others change theirs. I help overweight and obese adults reach their weight loss goals and gain confidence while they create a fit, healthy, energized lifestyle for themselves and their families.

Made in United States
Cleveland, OH
21 July 2025

18716851R00031